DK American College of Physicians

HOME MEDICAL GUIDE *to*

ASTHMA

D0822757

American College
of Physicians

HOME MEDICAL GUIDE *to*

ASTHMA

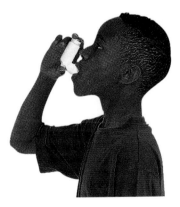

MEDICAL EDITOR
DAVID R. GOLDMANN, MD
ASSOCIATE MEDICAL EDITOR
DAVID A. HOROWITZ, MD

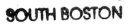

A DORLING KINDERSLEY BOOK

IMPORTANT

The American College of
Physicians (ACP) Home Medical
Guides provide general
information on a wide range of
health and medical topics. These
books are not substitutes for
medical diagnosis, and you should
always consult your doctor on
personal health matters before
undertaking any program of
therapy or treatment. Various
medical organizations have
different guidelines for diagnosis
and treatment of the same
conditions; the American College
of Physicians–American Society of
Internal Medicine (ACP–ASIM)
has tried to present a reasonable
consensus of these opinions.

Material in this book was
reviewed by the ACP–ASIM for
general medical accuracy and
applicability in the United States;
however, the information provided
herein does not necessarily reflect
the specific recommendations
or opinions of the ACP–ASIM.
The naming of any organization,
product, or alternative therapy in
these books is not an ACP–ASIM
endorsement, and the omission of
any such name does not indicate
ACP–ASIM disapproval.

DORLING KINDERSLEY

LONDON, NEW YORK, AUCKLAND, DELHI,
JOHANNESBURG, MUNICH, PARIS, AND SYDNEY

DK www.dk.com

Senior Editors Jill Hamilton, Nicki Lampon
Senior Designer Jan English
DTP Design Jason Little
Editor Irene Pavitt
Medical Consultant Gregory Tiro, MD

Senior Managing Editor Martyn Page
Senior Managing Art Editor Bryn Walls

Published in the United States in 2000 by
Dorling Kindersley Publishing, Inc.
95 Madison Avenue, New York, New York 10016

2 4 6 8 10 9 7 5 3 1

Library of Congress Catalog Card Number 99-76867
ISBN 0-7894-4162-4

Reproduced by Colourscan, Singapore
Printed and bound in the United States by Quebecor World, Taunton, Massachusetts

Contents

What is asthma?

Most people would recognize asthma in a child or an adult as attacks of wheezing and shortness of breath on exertion or at rest, sometimes mild and sometimes more severe. Some would recognize specific "triggers," such as animals, fumes, or pollens.

ASTHMA SYMPTOMS
A common symptom of asthma is wheezing, often with chest tightness and shortness of breath.

Some might think of asthma as a childhood condition, others as a condition that can affect someone of any age. Some would regard it as an occasional nuisance requiring intermittent treatment only, others as a persistent, significant problem that requires continuous treatment. Surely they can't all be right.

In a way, they are, although it is this wide range of factors involved in asthma that makes it extremely difficult to come up with a simple definition.

The word "asthma" is used as a blanket term to cover a condition that is characterized by episodes of shortness of breath caused by narrowing of the bronchial tubes, or the airways, within the lungs. There are many factors that contribute to the development of asthma and many that can induce attacks. In addition, these factors vary among individuals.

The Respiratory System

The airways (trachea, bronchi, and bronchioles) and airspaces within the lungs supply oxygen to and remove carbon dioxide from the body. Mucus is moved out of the lungs through the airways by cilia, or tiny hairs, on the airways' internal walls.

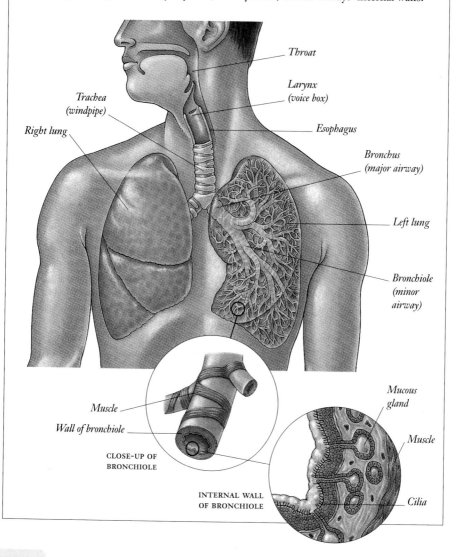

Throat

Larynx
(voice box)

Trachea
(windpipe)

Esophagus

Right lung

Bronchus
(major airway)

Left lung

Bronchiole
(minor
airway)

Muscle

Wall of bronchiole

CLOSE-UP OF
BRONCHIOLE

Mucous
gland

Muscle

Cilia

INTERNAL WALL
OF BRONCHIOLE

Asthma is best defined as a condition in which the airways within the lungs are inflamed and are therefore more sensitive to specific factors, or triggers, that cause them to narrow. This reduces airflow through the airways and makes the individual wheeze and feel short of breath. This sensitivity of the airways carries the medical label "bronchial hyperreactivity."

Asthma is not just one disease but covers a multitude of different patterns. Under this general heading, there are a range of severities, a range of triggering factors, and a range of outcomes. It logically follows that what is good for one asthmatic person may not be good for another.

Therefore, asthma is a very individual condition, and management needs to be personalized because of the variety of factors that underlie each individual's asthma.

KEY POINTS

- Asthma is not easy to define because of the wide range of factors that trigger it and the variety of airway responses it can cause.
- Asthma is not one disease but refers to a multitude of different patterns.

How common is asthma?

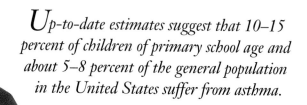

Up-to-date estimates suggest that 10–15 percent of children of primary school age and about 5–8 percent of the general population in the United States suffer from asthma.

Asthma is the most common condition in Western populations and affects more than 14.6 million adults and children in the US alone. In childhood, boys are affected twice as frequently as girls, while in adult life the condition is slightly more common among women than men. African–Americans are 26 percent more likely to suffer from asthma than are members of other ethnic groups.

CHILDHOOD ASTHMA
Asthma in children appears to be on the increase. Up to 20 percent of the school-aged population is believed to have asthmatic symptoms.

IS ASTHMA INCREASING?

Asthma has increased over the past two decades, regardless of what measure of asthma is considered. For example, between the mid-1970s and the early 1990s, there was about a fivefold increase in the number of patients visiting their doctors because of an asthma attack. There was also an increase in hospital admissions up to the early 1990s, particularly of children, possibly reflecting the fact that parents are more likely to seek medical advice for their children than for themselves. Fortunately, the rise stopped in the early 1990s and has even fallen slightly since then.

Why Did Asthma Increase?

It is possible that the increase in reported cases of asthma is partly due to doctors now using the word "asthma" more commonly than in the past, but this cannot explain most of the rise. Exposure to allergens in the home, viral infections, aspects of the indoor environment such as central heating, air pollution, the stress of modern living, and even the treatments used for asthma itself have all been blamed for the increase. However, evidence of any of these individual factors being entirely responsible is limited. In fact, it is very likely that the rise is due to a combination of these factors, although allergies are likely to be the most significant cause.

Deaths from Asthma

Fortunately, death from asthma is not common. In the mid-1960s a short-lived epidemic of deaths related to asthma occurred, which might have been the result of a toxic effect of one of the asthma inhalers available at the time. There has been some controversy over the years about this occurrence, and other factors may also have been important in these deaths, including the low socioeconomic status of the sufferers, many of whom lived in the inner cities and were members of minority ethnic groups; noncompliance with treatment; and the sufferers' episodic use of hospital emergency rooms rather than an established continuity of care with a doctor. It is unlikely that we shall ever know the complete story surrounding that particular event.

In fact, most deaths from asthma are caused by under-treatment of patients. It has been shown that two-thirds of asthma deaths might have been prevented by adequate treatment. More recently, there was a slight rise in asthma deaths in patients over the age of 50, although this stopped in the 1990s. Why this rise occurred is not clear, although differentiating between asthma and chronic bronchitis in older patients is often difficult, and it may have led to a change in diagnostic classification.

GEOGRAPHICAL DIFFERENCES

There are certainly some parts of the US where asthma admissions and visits to the doctor are more common and other areas where they are less so. However, the differences are modest and do not form a clear-cut geographical pattern, unlike attacks of acute bronchitis, which are higher in the North and lower in the South. Although the differences within the US are slight, there are large differences in the distribution of asthma in different parts of the world. Asthma is almost unheard of in Eskimos and sub-Saharan Africans living in rural areas, whereas in the Western Caroline Islands nearly 50 percent of the inhabitants have asthma, and 75 percent of the children are affected.

Between these two extremes are the Westernized populations, such as in the Americas, Europe, Australia,

ASTHMA-FREE POPULATIONS
Although asthma appears to be on the increase in many countries, there are places in the world where it is rare. For example, asthma rarely occurs among the Eskimo population of North America, possibly because the harsh climate is not hospitable to the house dust mite.

and New Zealand, which all have roughly the same prevalence of asthma. Interestingly, those parts of the world with the smallest number of asthma sufferers are those that are the least encouraging to the survival of the house dust mite.

KEY POINTS

- More than 14.6 million individuals in the United States have asthma.
- Boys are more frequently affected than girls, but the condition is slightly more common in women than in men, and African-Americans are 26 percent more likely to have asthma than are members of other ethnic groups.

Causes and triggers of asthma

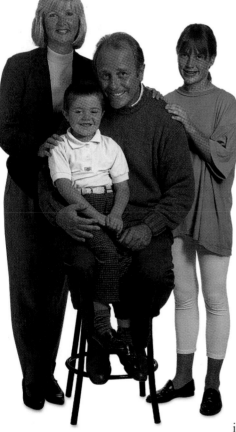

Most people know that asthma can run in families, and there is undoubtedly a hereditary component to this condition, particularly in allergic, or extrinsic, asthma. The genetic factor is much less marked in patients in whom allergy is not involved (intrinsic asthma).

HOW DOES IT START?

The tendency to develop asthma is not absolute. It is not inherited in the way that eye color and blood group are, and a patient with very severe asthma can have children who never develop the condition.

The role of environmental factors, such as allergens or exposure to smoking, is therefore prominent in the development and exacerbation of asthma. Nevertheless, it is clear that in order for the "seed" of asthma to germinate, the "soil" must be right.

A FAMILY CONCERN
Asthma, particularly when an allergen is involved, has a tendency to run in families.

HOUSE DUST MITE AND OTHER FACTORS

Many factors seem to be responsible for the first appearance of the symptoms of asthma. For instance, asthma that begins in adult life often seems to start following a cold or viral infection. Alternatively, exposure to a trigger in the workplace may be the initiating factor.

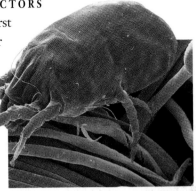

However, the most important factor in precipitating asthma, particularly in children, is exposure to the house dust mite. This little beast, smaller than a pinpoint, lives in our carpets, mattresses, furniture cushions, and furry toys. There can be as many as two million in each mattress.

When a susceptible individual is exposed to a protein in the fecal pellet of the house dust mite over a period of time, the body's white cells become sensitive to this foreign substance. As the protein is inhaled, a reaction to it occurs in the lining of the bronchial tubes, resulting in inflammation of the airways.

THE HOUSE DUST MITE
The feces of this mite (magnified here 500x), which lives in carpets, mattresses, and other furnishings, can trigger asthma.

The inflammation makes the lining irritable so that any further exposure, either to the house dust mite or any other trigger factor, will result in narrowing of the bronchial tubes and the symptoms of asthma.

There are other things that may be contributing factors to the initiation of asthma. Smoking by the mother during pregnancy and exposure to cigarette smoke in childhood may contribute in some cases.

The Development of Asthma

- Inheritance
- Mother smoking during pregnancy
- Exposure to cigarette smoke during childhood
- Allergens (especially the house dust mite)
- Colds or viral infections
- Occupational exposures

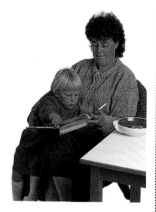

PASSIVE SMOKING
Exposure to other people's smoke is a contributory factor in childhood asthma. Smoking during pregnancy may also predispose a child to asthma.

AIRWAY INFLAMMATION

Asthma is a condition that causes inflammation and obstruction of the airways. Inflammation is the body's attempt to respond to a range of assaults; it can also be seen in many other illnesses, such as arthritis, colitis, and dermatitis. Problems arise for the patient when the inflammation does not clear up and becomes long-standing, or chronic, as is the case with asthma.

The normal airway is lined with a delicate protective layer called the mucosa, or epithelium. This layer consists of various types of cells with different functions. Some produce mucus, while others help clear the mucus from the airway by moving the secretions up the bronchial tubes by means of the movement of tiny fingers, or cilia, which are found on the surface of these cells. These cilia are some of the first structures to be destroyed by cigarette smoke, which also stimulates increased mucus production because the smoke causes inflammation. Smokers cough up phlegm as a result of this inflammation and of the increased mucus production that is caused. Cough is also a symptom in some patients with asthma. This is hardly surprising, since asthma is an inflammatory condition.

Below the mucosa, a second layer, the submucosa, lies over a spiral sheet of muscle that contracts when an asthmatic patient inhales a trigger such as grass pollen.

There are three separate processes that lead to airway narrowing and thus to wheezing and shortness of breath. First, the middle layer of the airway, or submucosa, becomes swollen; second, the mucous glands produce more secretions, which have to be coughed up to clear the airways; and third, the smooth muscle contracts as a result of the release of substances from inflammatory cells.

The net result of these three effects is narrowing of the airways, making it more difficult to get air in and out, which leads to wheezing and shortness of breath. Different forms of treatment have been devised to attack each component of airway narrowing.

In asthma, symptoms can occur for no obvious reason or may be caused by exposure to a known trigger factor, such as grass pollen. The airway narrowing can reverse itself, with improvement of symptoms, either spontaneously or following the use of a reliever drug. It is this variability that is so characteristic of asthma. Doctors take advantage of this not only when making the diagnosis but also when developing ways of keeping asthma under control and devising individual treatment regimens.

How Asthma Affects the Airways

During an asthma attack, the muscle walls of the airways (bronchi and bronchioles) contract, causing their internal diameter to narrow. Increased mucus secretion and inflammation of the airways' inner linings cause further narrowing.

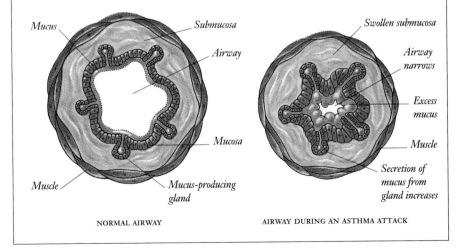

NORMAL AIRWAY

AIRWAY DURING AN ASTHMA ATTACK

CASE HISTORIES

If you have asthma you will already know that several factors can set off an attack (see chart on pp.20–21).

Case History 1: CHILDHOOD ASTHMA

John is seven years old. His mother, who had hay fever when she was younger, noticed that he had begun to cough when running around in the yard. She took him to the doctor, who prescribed antibiotics on three separate occasions. The antibiotics had no beneficial effect.

The symptoms became more persistent, and it was only when John started to wheeze whenever he exerted himself during recess at school that the connection was made, and a diagnosis of asthma followed. John now uses a bronchodilator (tube-opening) inhaler when he has symptoms. Since his diagnosis, John has been well and able to play without becoming short of breath.

Case History 2: FUR ALLERGY

Caroline, a 27-year-old woman with long-standing asthma, was referred to a chest specialist because of worsening symptoms over the previous two months. She had many allergic triggers for her asthma, including grass and tree pollens and a number of furry animals. Questions about her home life revealed that she was an avid cat lover with no fewer than 14 cats that she bred and exhibited at cat shows.

Caroline had an extremely strong skin-test reaction to cat fur but fervently denied that petting the cats made her worse. It was clear that the cats were a major cause of her continuing asthma, providing constant exposure to allergen and causing recurrent, almost continuous asthma episodes. She was not willing to get rid of the cats, and a

FURRY FRIENDS
Caroline's cats proved to be the main cause of her asthma attacks. She was allergic to their fur and dander (the dead skin that they constantly shed).

balance had to be struck between bad asthma caused by exposure to allergens and the benefits of keeping the cats.

Case History 3: PERFUME ALLERGY

Georgina had worked for 22 years in the cosmetics department of a department store. After a viral infection one autumn, she developed asthma, which initially was easy to treat with an inhaler as needed.

However, over the following year Georgina developed worsening symptoms, particularly cough, and the main trigger appeared to be scents. She stopped using perfumes herself, but, after an initial slight improvement, her symptoms clearly began to relate to her exposure to perfumes at the store. Eventually, she had to give up her job, and her symptoms improved immeasurably.

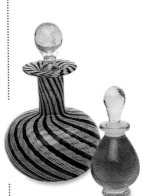

PERFUME SENSITIVITY
Georgina's sensitivity to perfumes began many years after she started work at a cosmetics department. Once sensitized, however, she could no longer tolerate contact with scents and had to leave her job.

Case History 4: AIR POLLUTION

David, a severe asthmatic in his 20s, had some difficulty controlling his asthma one autumn. He increased his inhaler usage, and his doctor prescribed two courses of steroid pills for him.

In the weeks before Christmas, David's asthma at last seemed to be stabilizing when a five-day air pollution episode hit the city, reaching peak levels on Christmas Eve. By that day, David's asthma had become much worse, and, in spite of more steroid pills and increased use of his nebulizer, he had to be admitted to the hospital.

Case History 5: POLLEN SENSITIVITY

One summer, a severe thunderstorm struck southern England, moving from the Southampton area, up through London and then northward through East Anglia.

Main Trigger Factors in Asthma

In a susceptible person, any of the following triggers can start an asthma attack.
An individual soon recognizes the factors that affect him or her.

EXERCISE

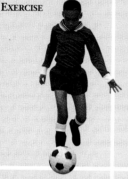

Exercise is a common trigger in children and may often be the only thing that brings on asthmatic symptoms. The problem is that shortness of breath on exertion is often attributed to weakness or not being in shape rather than to asthma. The child may then be perceived as not being strong enough to participate in sports or games with other children.

ALLERGENS

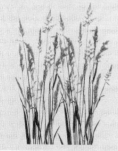

Pollen is the best-recognized trigger, but animals, particularly cats and horses, are also potent causes of attacks. Chronic exposure may result in more persistent symptoms. House pets may be missed as a trigger because the patient claims to be able to pet the animal without getting an attack, not realizing that long-term exposure is causing the chronic symptoms.

FUMES, DUST, AND ODORS

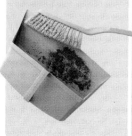

Cigarette smoke is a potent trigger for many patients, as are dusty environments, where the dust acts as an irritant. Odors, such as perfume or aftershave, can be a trigger for certain individuals, but this reaction is not an allergy. Presumably it is an irritant reaction to the chemicals involved, and the best treatment is avoidance whenever possible.

Main Trigger Factors in Asthma (cont'd.)

COLDS AND VIRUSES

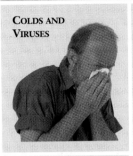

Viral infections are the most common trigger for asthma in people of all ages. Since antibiotics are effective only in treating bacterial infections, they should not be used routinely to treat colds due to viruses in patients with asthma. Not infrequently, however, a bacterial infection may follow a viral infection, in which case, antibiotics would be prescribed.

EMOTIONS AND STRESS

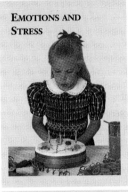

Children may often wheeze at birthday parties, where the combination of excitement and exertion makes asthma worse. For years, asthma was regarded as a neurotic condition, but we now know that emotional factors act only as triggers, not initiators, of asthma. Excitement, grief, and stress can all trigger an asthma attack.

CLIMATE AND POLLUTION

Many patients with asthma know that their condition is affected by the weather, but there is no uniform pattern. Some prefer cold to warm weather; others prefer hot, dry atmospheres. The patient usually knows best and will often adjust his or her behavior and treatment accordingly.

Air pollution episodes are well recognized as causing asthma attacks, particularly in patients with more severe asthma, in both the periods of high ozone levels during the summer and cold weather during the winter. There is, however, no direct evidence that exposure to air pollution at current levels will turn a nonasthmatic person into an asthmatic.

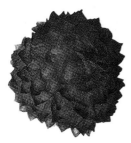

POLLEN GRAIN
*Seen here greatly
magnified, flower and
tree pollen grains can
trigger asthma attacks in
pollen-sensitive people.*

During this period, hundreds of patients went to emergency rooms with attacks of asthma. Many had no idea that they were asthmatic, although most admitted to wheezing with their hay fever. It is possible that a specific combination of meteorological factors and high pollen counts was the cause of the outbreak, a rather dramatic example of the weather affecting patients with asthma.

INTERACTING TRIGGER FACTORS

In many cases, two or more of these factors will interact, and different combinations will prove important for different individuals.

Asthma is a very personal condition. Consequently, what is good for one patient may not necessarily be good for another, and patterns of avoidance, treatment, and advance planning need to be determined for each person.

KEY POINTS

- Asthma can run in families, but a patient with severe asthma can have children who never develop the condition.
- The most important factor in initiating asthma, particularly in children, is the house dust mite.
- Symptoms may occur for no obvious reason or may be caused by exposure to one or more trigger factors, such as exercise, viral infection, fumes, dust, strong emotion, stress, climate, and pollution.
- Different combinations of trigger factors are important for different patients.

Symptoms and diagnosis

Diagnosis of asthma is often difficult because the symptoms can easily be confused with those of other respiratory complaints. A firm diagnosis may be made after a physical examination and specific tests.

A REASSURING TEST
Although a physical examination is reassuring, it is less important than tests of lung function.

▪ WHAT ARE THE SYMPTOMS? ▪

Asthma can occur with one or more of four main symptoms: wheezing, shortness of breath, cough, and chest tightness.

Wheezing and shortness of breath are the two best-recognized symptoms and usually come on intermittently in response to a known trigger or for no obvious reason. Both shortness of breath and wheezing can occur independently of each other.

One symptom often not recognized as being caused by asthma is cough, either a dry cough or a cough with sputum, which typically occurs at night or during exercise.

If the doctor fails to recognize that coughing can be caused by asthma, the condition may be misdiagnosed as

The Four Main Symptoms of Asthma

Wheezing and shortness of breath, the most common symptoms, may occur together or separately. Persistent cough is not as well recognized, and chest tightness may be apparent only during exertion.

WHEEZING
May occur with or without shortness of breath in response to a trigger or for no obvious reason.

SHORTNESS OF BREATH
Often associated with wheezing and coughing, but may also occur alone.

COUGHING
A sputum-producing or dry cough may be signs of asthma.

CHEST TIGHTNESS
Although often a symptom of asthma, chest tightness may be mistaken for a heart problem in older people.

bronchitis. Attacks of bronchitis are usually treated with antibiotics, which is an inappropriate treatment for asthma. More than two episodes of persistent cough, with or without wheezing or shortness of breath, should raise the question of underlying asthma in the minds of both doctor and patient.

The fourth main symptom of asthma is chest tightness. This often occurs during exertion, and, when an older person experiences chest tightness, a diagnosis of angina may be made. Thus, it might be a difficult problem for the doctor to diagnose asthma correctly.

Although the symptoms of asthma often occur for no apparent reason, they characteristically wake patients at night and are often a problem on waking in the morning. Waking up at night with asthma indicates that the asthma is being inadequately treated. Exercise and over-excitement, particularly in children, are frequent triggers for worsening symptoms.

— HOW IS ASTHMA DIAGNOSED? —

The trouble with these symptoms is that they occur in many other types of lung or heart conditions as well. A careful review of the symptoms – what sets them off, how long they last, how bad they are, and whether they show recognizable patterns – is necessary for the doctor to diagnose the condition accurately.

Although listening to the chest is part of any physical examination, very often it does not help the doctor a great deal when diagnosing an asthmatic person. The absence of wheezing does NOT mean that asthma is not the correct diagnosis.

EXERCISE AND ASTHMA
Children with asthma frequently find that exercise can precipitate an attack. However, if the asthma is adequately controlled, it should not be a barrier to sports and other activities.

25

Conditions That Share the Symptoms of Asthma

The symptoms of asthma occur in some other respiratory disorders and a few heart conditions. This table shows in which diseases and how commonly the symptoms are seen.

DIAGNOSIS	WHEEZING	SHORTNESS OF BREATH	COUGH	CHEST TIGHTNESS
Asthma	•••	•••	•••	•••
Chronic bronchitis	•••	•••	•••	••
Emphysema	••	•••	•	•••
Bronchiectasis	••	••	••••	••
Angina	•	••	•	••••
Heart failure	••	••••	••	••

KEY   • Symptom not usually seen   ••• Symptom often seen

•• Symptom can be seen   •••• Symptom virtually always seen

Conversely, not everyone who wheezes has asthma, making the diagnosis of asthma even more difficult.

BREATHING TESTS

Although asthma may be diagnosed on the basis of a medical history alone, some simple tests are often helpful. In older patients, in whom heart complaints are common, an electrocardiogram (ECG, or heart tracing) may be used to help evaluate for coronary artery disease, but breathing tests form the mainstay of asthma investigation.

There are two main types of breathing tests used in diagnosing asthma: peak flow tests and spirometry. Both measure how narrow the airways may be. The narrower the airways, the slower the flow of air through them and the lower the readings.

THE PEAK FLOW METER

The peak flow meter is a small, inexpensive instrument. It gives an idea of the narrowness of the airways by measuring the maximum, or peak, rate at which air can be expelled. This is the method most likely to be used by doctors as a single reading. However, you may be able to use one to measure your peak flow two, three, or four times a day to detect variation in values over the day. A person without asthma will show very little variation in peak flow over days or weeks, but an individual with asthma shows either consistent or intermittent variation. A common pattern is the "morning dip," in which the values are lowest on waking. Sometimes the fall in peak flow is intermittent, often in response to a recognized trigger such as cat fur.

Cursor

Scale (liters/minute)

Mouthpiece

PEAK FLOW METER
The peak flow meter is a simple device. After taking a deep breath, the user blows into the mouthpiece. The cursor is moved by the exhaled breath, and the point on the scale at which it comes to rest shows the maximum speed of air flow out of the lungs.

How to Use a Peak Flow Meter

Your doctor or nurse will show you how to use your peak flow meter correctly. These instructions are a reminder.

1 Stand up if possible.
2 Make sure cursor is at zero.
3 Take a deep breath, place peak flow meter in the mouth (hold horizontally), and close lips.
4 Blow suddenly and hard.
5 Note number indicated by cursor.
6 Return cursor to zero.
7 Repeat twice to obtain three readings.
8 Write down the best of the three readings.

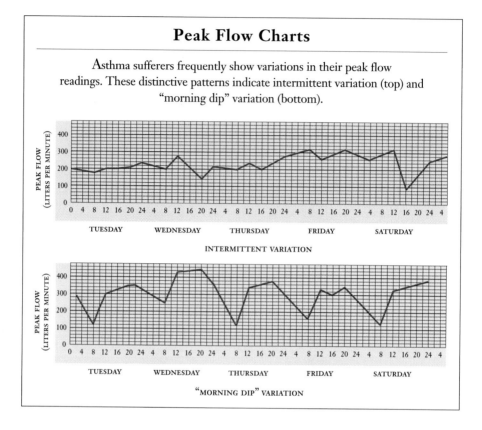

Peak Flow Charts

Asthma sufferers frequently show variations in their peak flow readings. These distinctive patterns indicate intermittent variation (top) and "morning dip" variation (bottom).

INTERMITTENT VARIATION

"MORNING DIP" VARIATION

Measuring peak flow in this way is particularly helpful if you experience symptoms only on an intermittent basis. Daily peak flow monitoring can be extremely helpful in management plans by acting as an early warning system to anticipate worsening asthma.

SPIROMETRY

Spirometry is used mostly by lung specialists and in hospitals, although an increasing number of primary care practitioners now use it as well. The test measures not only how fast air can be blown out but also the amount blown out with each breath. Spirometry provides more information but cannot give us the day-to-day measurements of peak flow readings.

REVERSIBILITY TESTS

Sometimes these breathing tests are performed before and after inhalation of a bronchodilator drug that opens the airways. If the readings increase by 15 percent or more after inhaling the drug, the airway narrowing is said to be reversible and confirms a diagnosis of asthma. Although asthmatic patients do not always show reversibility on every occasion tested, it is nevertheless a very useful diagnostic test in patients in whom asthma is suspected.

OTHER BREATHING TESTS

If your condition is difficult to diagnose, you may be sent to a pulmonary function laboratory, where more complicated tests can be performed.

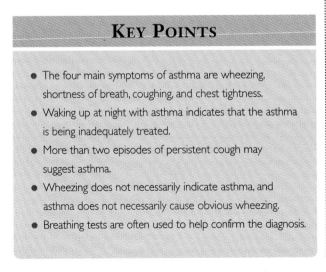

KEY POINTS

- The four main symptoms of asthma are wheezing, shortness of breath, coughing, and chest tightness.
- Waking up at night with asthma indicates that the asthma is being inadequately treated.
- More than two episodes of persistent cough may suggest asthma.
- Wheezing does not necessarily indicate asthma, and asthma does not necessarily cause obvious wheezing.
- Breathing tests are often used to help confirm the diagnosis.

Prevention and self-help

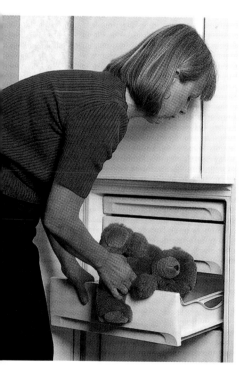

Although a diagnosis of asthma may seem to lead inevitably to the use of drugs to control the condition, there are several ways in which you and your family can help reduce symptoms. Equally, there are some environmental modifications that may be helpful.

— AVOIDING ALLERGENS —

Controlling the house dust mite can be very important to limiting asthma attacks in some patients, but measures to do so are expensive. The use of occlusive bedding is effective but extremely costly unless simple polyethylene sheeting is used to enclose the mattress and each pillow completely. Used alone, sprays to kill the mites are ineffective in controlling asthma. Ideally, carpets and slipcovers should be removed, and blinds should be used instead of curtains. Stuffed toys should be put in the freezer section of your refrigerator for 12 hours each week to kill the mites. Since these

MAKING STUFFED TOYS SAFE
Putting soft toys in the freezer compartment for 12 hours every week will kill house dust mites.

measures are time-consuming and expensive, inhalation therapy is a much easier way for most people to control their symptoms.

Getting rid of domestic pets is a contentious issue. Where there is undoubted allergy to cats, dogs, or rabbits, a balance has to be struck between controlling asthma by using inhalers and the grief that can be caused by banishing the pet. Nevertheless, long-term exposure to pets, even those that do not induce an obvious attack, can chronically worsen asthma by exposing a sensitized patient to high levels of allergen. In the more severely asthmatic patient, where control is more difficult, removal of the pet is mandatory.

Patients' wishes are very important. Some would rather get rid of a pet than use inhalers; others would prefer to suffer from asthma than lose what is often their best friend. Only when beliefs and wishes cause risk to the patient should the doctor be emphatic about parting with the family pet.

CENTRAL HEATING

There is no direct evidence that any particular form of central heating is either good or bad for patients with asthma. The belief that gas-fired central heating dries the air too much has been reported by some patients with asthma, but it is unlikely that this is a major problem. On the other hand, there are good theoretical reasons to believe that ducted or hot-air central heating may cause a problem, especially in those patients who are allergic

Helping Yourself or Your Child

- Don't smoke cigarettes
- Avoid "sick-contacts" wherever possible
- Control allergen exposures
- Establish a self-management plan with the help of your doctor
- Keep teachers informed about your child's asthma and the need for access to inhalers on demand
- Avoid known triggers

to the house dust mite. Unfortunately, it is very expensive to replace such heating systems, especially when there is no guarantee that the patient will improve afterward. However, if a new central heating system is being installed, it is probably best to avoid ducted or central hot-air systems if possible.

BEDROOM TEMPERATURE

A famous doctor of the seventeenth century, Sir John Floyer, himself an asthmatic, believed that when asthma woke a patient at night, it was due to "the heat of the bed." It has been said that sleeping with the bedroom window open, or at least keeping the air cool at night, may help people with asthma. In truth, there is no clear-cut answer. Some people prefer the cooler night air; other people find it causes them to wheeze more, particularly if they have to get up at night for some reason. It is up to you to adjust your environment according to whatever you find most effective.

COLDS AND FLU
Respiratory infections, such as the common cold or influenza, can cause asthmatic symptoms to worsen.

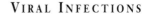

VIRAL INFECTIONS

Although viruses are an unavoidable cause of worsening asthma, it makes sense to avoid contact with someone who has an active cold. For schoolchildren, however, this is impractical. Children have to go to school and should not be kept home just because of the risk of catching a cold.

FOOD ALLERGIES

A small proportion of people with asthma, especially children, have food sensitivities. Again, a balance must be reached between the patient's wishes and the control of asthma. True food allergy is not particularly common but is undoubtedly more widespread than many doctors believe. The diagnosis of food allergy is often difficult and involves time-consuming tests. Skin tests can be misleading and should not be relied upon to diagnose or exclude food allergy. However, in an important minority, identifying a food or foods that worsen an individual's asthma can have a dramatic effect.

For example, a clear history of wheezing within minutes of eating a peanut is easy to recognize, and the best treatment is avoidance. On the other hand, sensitivity to dairy products or wheat is more difficult to recognize because the effects are more chronic and not as dramatic.

Case History 1: NUT ALLERGY

Nick had had asthma since childhood. He had always known that peanuts could cause very severe asthma attacks, but he had managed to prevent this by scrupulously avoiding all peanut-containing foods. During his teens Nick's asthma improved considerably, but he still avoided peanuts. On the rare occasion when he took in a mouthful of food containing peanuts, he immediately noticed a tingling sensation in his mouth and spat out the uneaten food. This usually prevented an attack.

One day, while eating a meal at the house of his new girlfriend, he suddenly realized the food that he had just swallowed contained peanuts. Within minutes, his tongue and lips became swollen and a severe asthma attack, known as anaphylactic shock, began. By the time he arrived at the hospital, he was blue and unconscious. Luckily, he got help in time, but he

A SEVERE REACTION
In some people, eating peanuts or food cooked with peanut oil may provoke a life-threatening asthmatic reaction.

still required mechanical ventilation for a short period before recovering. His girlfriend and her mother were distressed but had been unaware of his peanut allergy, one of the food allergies that patients rarely outgrow.

If you think you are sensitive to certain foods, you should consider consulting an allergist.

Case History 2: **WHEAT ALLERGY**

Carolyn was 35 years old and had had asthma since her teens. Initially it had affected her quality of life, but she had managed to develop a career and generally had her asthma under good control. Over a period of two to three years, however, Carolyn began to suffer worsening symptoms and found she needed frequent courses of oral steroids. She was referred to a specialist and drug treatment was increased to the maximum without success. She was then asked to undergo a food exclusion regimen; this testing suggested that she might be sensitive to wheat products. When tested with wheat in capsule form after a period of abstention, her asthma symptoms worsened over the next week, confirming the suspicion. Since avoiding wheat, Carolyn's asthma has been well controlled. She is still on inhalers at a moderate dose, but she has only rarely needed a course of oral steroids.

If you have a food allergy, not eating those foods is the only way to deal with the problem. Avoiding foods that are not often eaten, like shellfish, is relatively easy. However, if you are sensitive to certain dairy products or to wheat – two of the more commonly recognized problem foods – the restricted diet may become particularly

EXCLUSION DIET
Since eliminating wheat products such as bread from her diet, Carolyn's asthma has been well controlled.

tiresome and difficult to follow, especially if your asthma symptoms are modest. Some patients would prefer to stick to a restricted diet than take drugs. Only rarely, however, will asthma symptoms be completely controlled by dietary means.

CIGARETTE SMOKE

Cigarette smoke is bad for asthma. Fifteen to 20 percent of patients with asthma smoke, and these patients are more likely to end up hospitalized with acute asthma. Many cigarette smokers also often develop irreversible narrowing of their airways.

If you smoke, you must try to stop by whatever means you can. This may require a great deal of help from relatives and friends. "Just one" *will* hurt, and offering you a cigarette is a far from friendly act. There are a number of new and fairly successful smoking cessation strategies and medications. Your doctor can often assist you in finding appropriate treatment to help you stop.

Inhaling secondhand smoke causes considerable suffering in asthmatic children. The children of parents who smoke are more likely to have episodes of wheezing and school absences than are children of nonsmoking parents. This effect is most obvious when both parents smoke, but maternal smoking appears to be a greater problem than paternal smoking, in large part because most children usually spend more time with their mothers.

Smoking while you are pregnant will

BREAKING THE HABIT
Any smoker who suffers from asthma should give up smoking immediately. Asthmatics should also avoid smoky atmospheres.

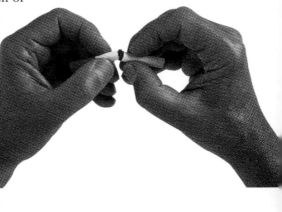

increase the risk of the child being born with asthma, even when taking into account other risk factors such as family history.

GAMES AND SCHOOL

Exercise-induced asthma is common in children and can cause other problems. Teachers may accuse kids of "not trying" or attempting to avoid sports, and their own schoolmates may tease them for "being useless." Sensible preparation can help. It is always a good idea for an asthmatic child to use a relief inhaler about 15 minutes before going out to play. If it is used immediately before he or she starts to play, the asthma symptoms will develop before the inhaler has a chance to work.

In some children, after the first episode of wheezing with exercise, there often follows a period when they can run and play for a long time without problems. Sometimes, this so-called refractory period has the unfortunate effect of reinforcing to a skeptical teacher or class-mate that the child was just trying to get out of gym.

Many teachers may be somewhat uninformed about asthma, although most are very eager to know more if they are offered the chance. If you have an asthmatic child, you should tell your child's teachers about the need for your son or daughter to have ready access to an inhaler.

All too often we hear of inhalers being locked away in the school secretary's office, which may be some distance from the playground. Explaining to your child's teachers how to allow the use of a relief inhaler without

SCHOOL GAMES
A relief inhaler used 15 minutes before any activity can help prevent wheezing.

permitting its abuse will dispel the teacher's concerns about the perceived dangers of inhalers.

SPORTS

Many top athletes have asthma and are able to compete at the highest level. Some of the self-help advice given above for children is applicable to adults, particularly in the use of inhalers before exercise. A warm-up period may help with the problem of exercise-induced symptoms to some extent, particularly before the first exercise of the day.

KEY POINTS

- Controlling house dust mites is important for some patients.
- Severe asthma may necessitate parting with a pet.
- Patients with food allergy can rarely completely control their asthma symptoms by dietary means alone.
- Asthmatic patients who smoke must stop.
- Smoking during pregnancy increases the risk of the child being born with asthma.
- Parents of an asthmatic child may need to explain to teachers the need for their child to have ready access to his or her inhaler.

Drugs used in the treatment of asthma

The drugs used in the treatment of asthma can be divided into three main groups: relievers, preventers, and emergency or reserve drugs.

A wide range of drugs are used to treat asthma, but they all fall into one of three groups depending on whether they relieve asthmatic symptoms or prevent them.

RELIEVERS

Relievers act by relaxing the muscle in the walls of the airways, allowing the airways to open up and air to get in and out more easily, thereby making breathing easier. These are called bronchodilator drugs and are given in inhaled form, dispensed by a small plastic inhaler. Inhalers come in a wide range of different types. They are most commonly used when symptoms occur rather than on a regular basis, but, if you have more severe asthma, your doctor may advise regular use.

PREVENTERS

These drugs act by reducing the inflammation in the airways, thus calming their irritability. In contrast to reliever inhalers, preventers must be taken on a regular basis, usually twice a day. It can be easy to forget to take

ASTHMA DRUGS
Inhalers provide a convenient way of getting drugs deep into the lungs.

Inhalation of Asthma Drugs

Inhaling an asthma drug is the most effective treatment for the prevention and relief of asthma. The inhaler distributes the drug rapidly through the airways for instant relief of symptoms.

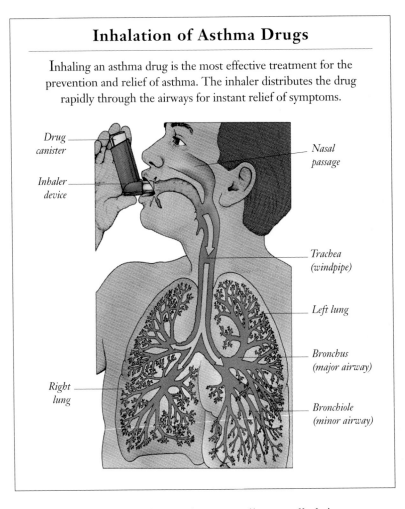

Drug canister

Inhaler device

Nasal passage

Trachea (windpipe)

Left lung

Bronchus (major airway)

Right lung

Bronchiole (minor airway)

the preventer inhaler when asthma is well controlled and symptoms are few and far between. Consequently, many patients keep the preventer inhaler next to their toothbrush as a reminder. There are three main types of preventer drug: inhaled steroids, cromolyn sodium, and nedocromil sodium. These come in a variety of inhaler devices (see pp.79–86).

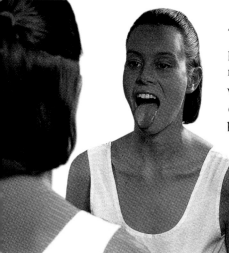

INHALED STEROIDS

The word "steroid" conjures up disturbing pictures in many people's minds, and there is much misinformation circulating about these very effective drugs.

- Inhaled steroids are not the anabolic type used by bodybuilders and, illegally, by some athletes.

  - The inhaled version used as preventive treatment is the same sort of drug as steroid pills used for acute attacks of asthma and in some patients with arthritis.

  - The dose of the inhaled drug is very small compared with that contained in steroid pills. For example, in acute asthma, six 5-milligram pills of steroid may be given per day – 30,000 micrograms of drug, which is 75 times a typical inhaled daily dose of approximately 400 micrograms of drug.

- The side effects of inhaled steroids are few compared to those of oral steroids but, most importantly, they are very much less dangerous than undertreated asthma.

- Of the patients on inhaled steroids, 5 percent will complain of a sore or dry mouth (sometimes this is due to an oral yeast infection), and another 5 percent may complain of some huskiness in their voice. This side effect is more bothersome to patients who use their voice a lot, such as teachers or telemarketers.

- At higher doses (1,500 micrograms per day or more), particularly in older patients, side effects such as bruising easily may become apparent, along with an increase in the frequency of oral yeast infections and hoarseness. Cataracts may occur in some patients, but

SIDE EFFECTS
A few patients will experience a sore or dry mouth when taking inhaled steroids. This may be due to an oral yeast infection. If you experience this, check your throat in the mirror, and see your doctor if you think there is any cause for concern.

The Main Types of Asthma Drug

- Relievers
- Preventers
- Emergency/reserve drugs

the suggestion that inhaled steroids cause osteoporosis (thinning of the bones) is debatable. Any such effects have to be balanced against the risks of asthma if it is under-treated. The local effects of these inhalers can be minimized by rinsing the mouth after each dose and by using large-volume spacer devices such as Aerochambers (see pp.45–46). These devices act as "reservoirs" and thereby reduce the amount of medication that is deposited in the mouth.

● There is some evidence that a small proportion of children may show slight growth suppression with high doses of inhaled steroids but, interestingly, once the asthmatic child reaches adult height, normal growth virtually always resumes. Chronic, under-treated asthma in childhood is more likely to cause growth suppression than are inhaled steroids.

Inhaled steroids are very effective preventive drugs across the full spectrum of patients with asthma and are regarded as the preventive treatment of choice in most of these patients.

CROMOLYN SODIUM

Cromolyn sodium has been available for as long as inhaled steroids have been. It is a very good form of prevention in milder forms of childhood asthma, particularly in controlling exercise-induced symptoms. It should be used three or four times a day, a disadvantage

The Main Types of Preventer Drug

Preventer drugs are used on a regular basis to control and minimize symptoms of asthma. This table shows the three main types of inhaled preventer drugs.

- Inhaled steroids
- Cromolyn sodium
- Nedocromil sodium

when compared with inhaled steroids, but it can be used simply before exercise to prevent exercise-induced symptoms and has virtually no side effects.

NEDOCROMIL SODIUM

Nedocromil sodium has a preventive effect comparable to that of low-dose inhaled steroids and comes as a mint-flavored dry powder aerosol.

OTHER PREPARATIONS

There are two other groups of drugs used in the treatment of asthma. These are the theophyllines and the new leukotriene inhibitors.

• Theophylline is available in various brand-name products, which were originally used as bronchodilators but tend to be used more in a preventive way now. They are probably used less now than in the past because of the effectiveness and safety of inhaled steroids. They tend to cause nausea and headache in some patients but have the advantage of being available in pill form, which is especially useful for people who have difficulty using an inhaler.

• The leukotriene inhibitors (zafirlukast, zileuton, and montelukast) are a completely new form of asthma treatment. They are essentially preventive drugs but they do have slight bronchodilator effects. Since they have only recently been approved, it has not yet been determined which patients may be best treated with these drugs. However, they are particularly effective for patients with aspirin-sensitive asthma and may prove to be the treatment of choice for these people. So far, leukotriene inhibitors seem to have relatively few side effects.

The Main Types of Inhaled Asthma Drugs

The majority of asthma drugs are inhaled. They may be relievers, which ease the symptoms once an attack has started, or preventers, which are used regularly to keep asthma under control.

RELIEVERS		PREVENTERS	
GENERIC NAME	BRAND NAME	GENERIC NAME	BRAND NAME
Albuterol	Ventolin Proventil	Beclomethasone (50, 100, 200, 250, 400 mcg)	Beclovent Vanceril
Salmeterol xinafoate	Serevent	Budesonide	Pulmicort 200 mcg (including Turbohaler)
Ipratropium bromide	Atrovent		
Albuterol sulfate & ipratropium bromide	Combivent	Fluticasone propionate	Flovent 44, 110, 220 mcg
Pirbuterol acetate	Maxair	Triamcinolone acetonide	Azmacort
Metaproterenol sulfate	Alupent	Flunisolide	Aerobid
		Cromolyn sodium	Intal (puffer 5 mcg) (spincaps 20 mcg)
		Nedocromil sodium	Tilade

EMERGENCY TREATMENT

When an acute attack of asthma occurs, there are two mainstays of emergency treatment available: high doses of reliever drug (often delivered by a nebulizer) and high doses of an anti-inflammatory drug (injected or taken in the form of oral steroids).

Some patients who have an acute attack will be able to start emergency treatment themselves with a nebulizer and/or oral steroids, but most patients who have not had a severe attack before should contact their doctor as quickly as possible or go to the emergency room of the local hospital. Delay can be very dangerous, and it is better to be safe than sorry.

The nebulized drug used most commonly in acute episodes is albuterol. A nebulizer should be obtained only after your asthma has been assessed by a doctor. The machine itself is a simple air compressor that bubbles air through a solution of the drug, generating a mist that is inhaled through a mask or a plastic mouthpiece.

In some cases, nebulized drugs may be prescribed for regular use by the more severely asthmatic patient, but only in cases when high doses of other treatments have proved to be inadequate.

Nebulizers should not be used instead of inhaled preventive treatment.

USING A NEBULIZER
The nebulizer is a simple air compressor. It bubbles air through a drug solution, generating a mist that is inhaled through either a mouthpiece or a mask.

How Drugs Act on Blocked Airways

Preventer drugs and reliever drugs act in different ways. Preventers reduce the inflammation in the airways, thus calming their irritability. Relievers act by relaxing the muscles in the walls of the airways, allowing the airways to open up.

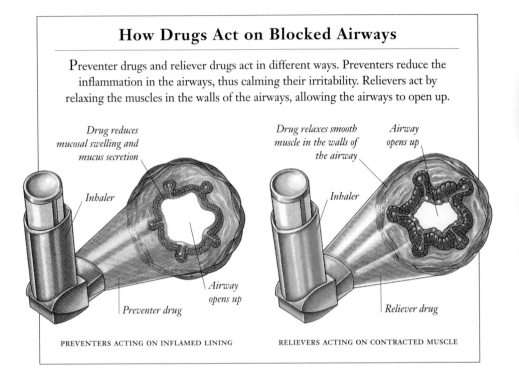

Drug reduces mucosal swelling and mucus secretion

Inhaler

Airway opens up

Preventer drug

Drug relaxes smooth muscle in the walls of the airway

Airway opens up

Inhaler

Reliever drug

PREVENTERS ACTING ON INFLAMED LINING

RELIEVERS ACTING ON CONTRACTED MUSCLE

DELIVERY DEVICES

Many patients cannot use simple metered dose inhalers (puffers) effectively. Poor inhalation technique can result in the drug escaping from the inhaler into the air.

The patient then believes that the inhaler is not working properly, when it has not been given a chance to work at all. If you are one of these patients, you can use another type of inhaler device that relies on your breath for sucking the drug into your lungs, rather than the puffer, with which your inhaling has to coincide with the squirt of the puffer.

The most frequently used type of breath-activated device is the spacer, a plastic tube that serves as a reservoir of drug from the puffer for the patient to breathe in at the right moment. Spacers are made of rigid plastic, and there is some evidence that they can acquire a lot of static electrical charge. This static electricity causes the medication to stick to the inside of the spacer, thereby reducing the amount of drug getting into the lungs. The best strategy is to wash the spacer once a week and allow it to drip dry. Rubbing the spacer with an antistatic cloth can also help reduce this problem.

USING A SPACER
If you have to give drugs for asthma to small children, you may find it easier to use a reservoir device such as this spacer. With devices, the child does not have to inhale at the same time as the puffer is pressed.

Other types of breath-activated devices include Rotahalers, Turbohalers, Spinhalers, and Autohalers, all of which have their benefits and shortcomings (see pp.79–86). In many cases, it is clear that an individual patient feels most comfortable with a particular device.

Matching the patient with the right type of inhaler is vital. An acceptable device is more likely to be used effectively and at the correct time and frequency. With the exception of the spacer devices, breath-activated inhalers are the most expensive. However, an expensive device that is used correctly may in the long run be less expensive in terms of patient suffering than a poorly used "bargain" device.

▪ CHLOROFLUOROCARBON INHALERS ▪

Metered dose inhalers, or puffers, contain chlorofluorocarbons (CFC) as a propellant. Because of the effect of CFCs on the ozone layer, puffers containing CFCs should be phased out. Some puffers that contain an alternative propellant have already been released; others will be on the market this year. They look similar to existing puffers but tend to have a more noticeable taste. However, the drug in each inhaler is the same, and they are just as effective.

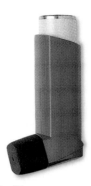

THE METERED DOSE INHALER
This device, commonly known as a "puffer," is used to deliver fast-acting reliever drugs. Some people, particularly children, find it difficult to use.

KEY POINTS

- Drugs used in asthma treatment are relievers, preventers, and emergency reserve drugs.
- Inhaled steroids are the preventive treatment of choice for most patients with asthma.
- The right combination of drug and inhaler device needs to be chosen for each patient.

The management of asthma

The goal of managing asthma is to put you, the patient, in control of your asthma rather than letting the asthma control your life.

For patients who require only an occasional puff of their relief inhaler, control of asthma is easy. For patients with more significant asthma, guidelines need to be developed and agreed upon by doctor and patient. Asthma is a very personal condition, and what is right for one person may not be right for another. There are, nevertheless, guidelines that have recently been developed to help doctors and nurses in the management of all asthmatic patients. The guidelines were developed by a panel of experts representing the different groups involved in the management of asthma.

The guidelines are simple to follow. They are based on a series of upward steps to control asthma and a series of downward steps when asthma appears to be in good control and when lower levels of treatment may be sufficient.

JOINT MANAGEMENT
Doctor and patient should formulate a management plan together in order to establish good control of asthma.

Preventive measures, similar to those that are discussed in Prevention and self-help (see pp.30–37), include control of allergens. It is very important to avoid certain drugs that cause asthma or make it worse (such as aspirin or beta blockers). You should stop taking these medications if you begin to develop wheezing and shortness of breath, even if you have been using them for some time without problems. You should also stop drugs similar to aspirin and seek alternatives (see Special forms of asthma, pp.60–66).

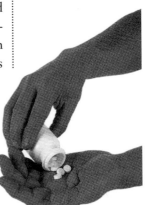

GUIDELINE STEPS

The following guidelines are the National Asthma Guidelines of the National Institutes of Health, which have recently been updated. They employ a graded method of controlling asthma symptoms using the minimum amount of medication.

FINDING ALTERNATIVES
Some medications such as aspirin can cause or exacerbate asthma. Stop taking medications that precipitate wheezing, and consult your doctor about alternatives.

Step 1 (Mild Intermittent) Most patients are at this level. Patients are advised to use their relief inhalers as required. If your use of the relief inhaler stays at less than twice per week and you have nighttime symptoms less than twice per month, no further drug treatment need be considered. If you are using one regularly more than twice per week, contact your doctor about moving to Step 2.

Step 2 (Mild Persistent) If, on average, you are using your relief inhaler more than twice per week but less than once a day or have nighttime symptoms more than twice per month, you need a preventive inhaler. As a general rule, the choice is made by the doctor (see Drugs used in the treatment of asthma, pp.38–47) and it will be prescribed at a low dose. This should allow you to reduce your use of an inhaled reliever to less than twice a week and should improve your symptoms.

Step 3 (Moderate Persistent) If on average you have daily symptoms requiring use of an inhaler; if exacerbations occur twice or more per week, last days at a time, and inhibit activity; or if nighttime symptoms occur more than once a month, you are likely to need more aggressive inhaled therapy. This may include medium-dose inhaled steroids or low- to medium-dose inhaled steroids with a long-acting inhaled beta-agonist or sustained-relief theophylline. These decisions are made by the doctor in consultation with you and after assessment of your particular needs.

Step 4 (Severe Persistent) If you have continual symp toms, limited physical activity because of your asthma, frequent exacerbations, or frequent nighttime symptoms, then the use of even higher doses of inhaled preventive treatment, oral steroid use, and nebulizers, among other treatment options, will be considered. At this stage it is likely that you will be referred to a pulmonary specialist for assessment.

Step down It may sometimes be too easy to start a new treatment when symptoms do not come under control. It is not as easy to stop a treatment either when symptoms are well controlled or when a new drug has had no extra benefit.

MANAGEMENT PLANS

One way of having control over your asthma and its treatment is through a management plan. This is a

Steps to Asthma Control

These simple guidelines, developed by doctors and nurses involved in the treatment of asthma, allow for the minimum dose of the appropriate drug to be given so that the symptoms are adequately controlled.

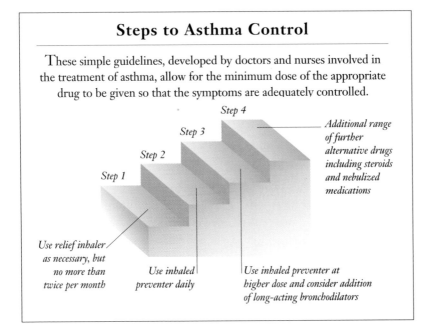

Step 1

Step 2

Step 3

Step 4

Additional range of further alternative drugs including steroids and nebulized medications

Use relief inhaler as necessary, but no more than twice per month

Use inhaled preventer daily

Use inhaled preventer at higher dose and consider addition of long-acting bronchodilators

series of instructions that explain what you should do when your asthma gets worse or in situations in which your asthma might become worse. There are two types of management plans.

PEAK FLOW-BASED MANAGEMENT PLANS

The peak flow meter is simple to use. A short, strong effort will indicate the maximum rate at which you can blow air out of your lungs. Usually, you make three attempts and record the highest one. Recording a value twice a day, on waking and on going to bed, is usually sufficient, although sometimes your doctor will ask for more frequent readings.

With a peak flow-based management plan, you are provided with a peak flow meter, a chart on which you will record the peak flow readings, and target peak flow values.

A key value is the target peak flow, which is usually 70–80 percent of the optimal value predicted according to one's age, size, and gender. If your peak flow is above this value, you do not need to adjust your treatment. If your peak flow falls below this level over a 24-hour period, you should double your normal inhaled preventive treatment until your peak flows have climbed above the target peak flow and remained there for two or three days.

If your peak flow falls to a second threshold of about 50–60 percent of your predicted value, you should use oral steroids.

You may be allowed to take this course of action yourself, but some doctors prefer to see the patient if oral steroids are needed.

A final threshold is that at which you should seek medical assistance as soon as possible, from either your doctor or the local emergency room. This level of peak flow will be set by the doctor.

The chart for recording peak flows may be either a series of columns on which the recordings are written, usually twice a day, or a graphlike chart to plot the values. Some patients prefer this second type of chart because the variation in levels of peak flow can be more easily seen and understood.

Case History 1: **PEAK FLOW-BASED PLAN**

Bill had always been a difficult boy, and not just as far as his asthma was concerned. He tended to use his inhalers only when he felt the need and consequently was constantly missing school. By the time he had reached middle school, his asthma had not improved, and his doctor decided to try to establish a management plan.

For the first time, Bill started to record his peak flow readings at home when he woke up in the morning and at night before he went to bed. The peak flow meter stayed by his bed, and his parents were able to check that he was recording the values on his chart. Somewhat to his surprise, Bill found that his peak flow readings varied considerably, dropping as low as 150 on waking but reaching 270 by evening.

Now that he could make the connection himself, Bill began to take his inhaled preventive medication more regularly. The peak flow variation became less marked, and the readings also increased somewhat, averaging between 300 and 350. By that stage, Bill was taking two puffs of inhaled steroid morning and night and needed to use the relief inhaler much less frequently.

The doctor then gave him a target of 275, advising him to double his preventer dosage if the values dropped below this level over a 24-hour period and to stay at the higher dose until he was above the peak-flow target for at least three days.

A second threshold was given of 175, below which Bill knew to contact his doctor for oral steroids. In fact, oral steroids never became necessary. Bill began to notice the benefits of his regular preventive therapy. Over the subsequent year he had to increase his inhaled steroids, when peak flows fell below 275, on only three occasions.

SYMPTOM-BASED MANAGEMENT PLANS

This plan is similar to a peak flow-based plan, but certain levels of symptoms, rather than changes in peak flow, are used as prompts for changes in treatment.

| Case History 2: **SYMPTOM-BASED PLAN** |

Jackie had not done well with peak flow measurements. They did not seem to tell her much more about her asthma than did her symptoms, and they began to be a nuisance to do. She felt that she was doing it "just for the sake of the doctor," as she saw it. Fortunately, the doctor became aware of this and suggested a switch to a symptom-based plan. By doubling her inhaled preventive dose if she used more than three puffs of relief inhaler a day over two successive days, if she caught a cold, or if she woke at night with symptoms, her asthma was more effectively controlled. If doubling the inhaled preventer did not stop her symptoms, Jackie knew that she had to go to her doctor for reassessment. In that case she measured her peak flow a few times before going. This helped her manage her asthma sensibly.

CHOOSING A PLAN

Some patients seem better suited to peak flow-based plans, and others to symptom-based plans. The decision of which plan to use is often based on a number of factors. Sometimes a combination of symptoms and peak flow can be used for certain individuals. Both plans include advice to anticipate problems such as colds or exposure to known allergens. If you develop the early symptoms of a cold, you should double your inhaled preventive treatment for at least a week until the symptoms pass, and then resume the original dose. Some patients need inhaled steroids only for colds. They should start at the first hint of a cold and continue for two weeks. If their asthma continues to cause problems, they should stay on the preventive treatment and contact the doctor.

CLINICS

Asthma clinics have been set up in many doctors' offices, run either by the doctor or a technician. Many are run by physicians specifically trained in the management of asthma. Their role is very important, and they have helped provide much better service for asthmatic patients. There have been fewer referrals to the hospital from offices or clinics with such a system and more appropriate referrals when there are problems.

Often, the nurse or technician will see patients with asthma more frequently than the doctor does, but they know when the doctor needs to see the patient if things are not going well. It should be the goal of all primary care practices to set up or provide access to an asthma clinic run by a fully-trained associate or technician.

KEY POINTS

- Guidelines have been developed to help doctors and nurses provide optimal management of all asthmatic patients using a series of treatment steps.
- One way of giving patients good control over their asthma is to provide them with a management plan.
- Management plans may either be peak flow-based or symptom-based.
- Many doctors have set up asthma clinics, often run by specially trained associates or technicians.

Asthma in the elderly

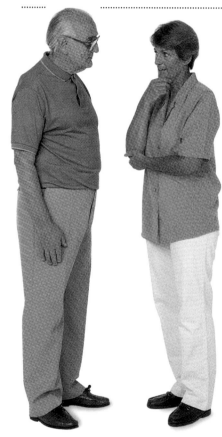

Asthma tends to be seen as a condition of the young, and it is indeed much more common in children. As these patients grow older, some have persistent problems, some have only minor symptoms, and some have none.

Some patients develop asthma for the first time in their later years. It is often believed that these patients are more likely to have more severe asthma and to need oral steroids. It has also been suggested that allergies are less likely to be a contributing factor. While these beliefs are true up to a point, it is important to realize that there is a great overlap of asthma patterns in every age group. Each patient must be assessed as an individual.

LATE DEVELOPMENT
Although asthma is much more common in children and the young, it can persist or even begin in later life.

SYMPTOMS

Symptoms in older patients are nearly identical to those found in younger patients with asthma. However, shortness of breath, especially on exertion, is more common.

This is often due to the fact that many people over the age of 60 have at some time in their lives smoked cigarettes and are left with some degree of irreversible bronchial tube narrowing. Exertion will cause shortness of breath more quickly in those individuals who have smoked in the past because of the bronchial narrowing.

Problems can occur when an older patient complains of chest tightness on exertion. Since heart disease is common in this age group and angina can cause this very same symptom, delay in diagnosis of either angina or asthma can occur.

Case History: LATE-ONSET ASTHMA

Tom, an 82-year-old man, went to his doctor with a six-month history of episodes of shortness of breath. Sometimes these came on without warning, and sometimes they happened when he exerted himself. He did not feel that he was wheezing but did admit that he had a tight feeling in his chest, particularly when he became short of breath on exertion.

The doctor's first impression was that, in a gentleman of this age, the shortness of breath might to be due to heart disease, but treatment for angina had no effect. Tom was sent to a specialist who felt that late-onset asthma needed to be ruled out, although he was fairly certain that this was an unlikely diagnosis. To the specialist's surprise, the peak flow readings that were assiduously recorded recorded by the patient showed the typical variation seen in asthma, and prescription of antiasthma medication, after confirmation of the diagnosis with formal spirometry and pulmonary function testing, resulted in great improvement in his symptoms. However, the patient's reaction when he heard that he had asthma was one of anger.

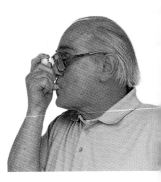

INVESTIGATING SYMPTOMS
Shortness of breath in the elderly is often caused by heart disease, and symptoms should always be investigated in this group. In Tom's case, peak flow measurements showed that he was suffering from late-onset asthma. Inhaled antiasthma medication relieved his symptoms.

"Why me? I've never smoked and I've always looked after myself. There's no one in the family who has suffered from asthma. Why me?"

His anger abated in response to the doctor's explanation and reassurance, and to the fact that on two puffs of inhaled steroid twice a day he improved greatly. He is now able to garden as he did before with only occasional need to use his relief inhaler.

WHAT IS THE TREATMENT?

Treatment of asthma in the older patient is the same and follows the same steps as in the younger patient. Problems can occur, however, in using the inhaler devices. The Rotacap dry powder system can be difficult for an arthritic hand, and even the metered dose inhaler (puffer) can be impossible for patients with stiff or painful hands. A large-volume spacer, such as that used for children (see pp.45–46), will often solve the problem. It is really a matter of tailoring the inhaler device to the patient.

As patients age, they often find themselves on a variety of different pills and other medications for a range of conditions. This can often be very confusing, and it is the doctor's responsibility to keep the regimen of treatment as simple as possible. It may even be necessary to sacrifice the ideal treatment just to make sure that the most important treatments are taken.

Side effects from any form of treatment are more common in older patients. In more severe asthmatics, the side effects of oral steroids can be acute, with easy bruising, skin thinning, and poor wound healing. Patients taking high-dose inhaled steroids (more than 1,500 micrograms per day) can also develop these side effects, although to a less dramatic degree.

WHAT IS THE OUTLOOK?

As mentioned earlier, deaths from asthma have increased in elderly people over the past five to ten years, but the reasons for this trend are not clear. One explanation is that, formerly, many such people would have been thought to have died of bronchitis. Indeed, although some of these deaths from asthma may be due more to chronic bronchitis, doctors must not be complacent in their attempts to prevent death from asthma at whatever age it causes problems.

The treatment of asthma at any age is safe and effective, although people who are severely affected may need to find a balance between the symptoms of their asthma and the side effects of drugs.

KEY POINTS

- Asthma can develop later in life, and older sufferers are more prone to shortness of breath, especially on exertion.
- Angina and asthma can be difficult to differentiate in the elderly.
- Side effects of asthma treatment are more common in older patients.
- Although the asthma is unlikely to go away, elderly sufferers can enjoy effective control of their symptoms with proper treatment targeted to their individual needs.

Special forms of asthma

In many cases, the cause of asthma is unknown. In others, however, an allergen will commonly trigger an attack. Other special forms of asthma include life-threatening asthma, aspirin-sensitive asthma, and nocturnal asthma.

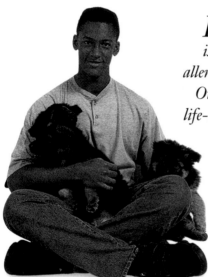

IDENTIFYING ALLERGENS
If you suspect that your asthma is caused by a particular allergen, such as cats or dogs, it can be confirmed by a special allergy test.

ALLERGIC ASTHMA

If an allergy (or more than one allergy) has been identified as being potentially important on the basis of your history, it is sometimes necessary to take additional tests to confirm and identify the allergen(s). The test is simple and takes about half an hour to complete.

A series of drops of various solutions of substances known to cause allergic reactions (such as the house dust mite, grass pollen, tree pollen, and cat dander) are placed on the forearm. Using small needle points, the skin surface is gently pierced through each droplet to allow the substance to get under the skin. Local reactions, which look like small areas of rash and usually itch, can occur 15 minutes or so after the test is administered. The needle pricks themselves are uncomfortable

Some Potential Triggers of Allergy

Asthma allergens enter the body through a variety of routes. They can be inhaled, eaten, or absorbed through the skin. Some of the most common allergens are shown here.

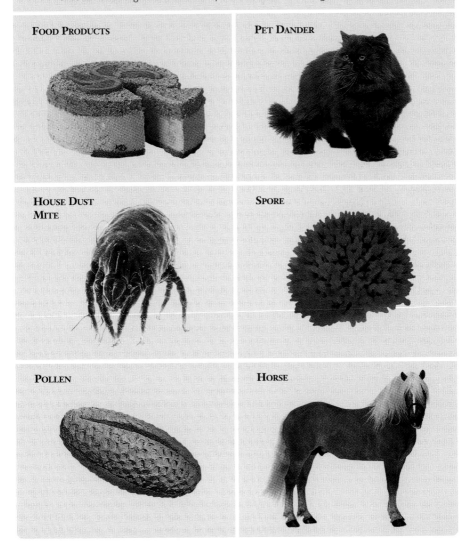

FOOD PRODUCTS

PET DANDER

HOUSE DUST MITE

SPORE

POLLEN

HORSE

but not painful, but the itching can be intense and lasts half an hour or so.

The size of the reaction (or wheal) for each allergen can be measured. It gives an idea not only of what you are allergic to but also how allergic you may be to each allergen. Sometimes this is helpful in management because it can tell you which triggers to avoid and which are not as important.

Minor reactions may not be very important, but some patients may take unnecessary precautions to avoid them. The occasional patient may follow extraordinary and unnecessary diets, based on only weakly positive skin tests, and find that they are not helpful.

DESENSITIZATION

If you are shown to be allergic to a particular allergen, such as cat or rabbit dander, you cannot avoid contact with these animals, and your asthma continues to be poorly controlled by the usual treatment regimens, desensitization may be considered. Great care must be taken for those patients who have asthma, however, and the tests and treatment should be conducted only at a hospital or where emergency care is available because there have been many cases of severe reactions to desensitization, from asthma attacks that require hospital admission to sudden death. For those patients who only have hay fever, the danger is much less.

The desensitization process involves a series of injections of small amounts of the substance to which you are allergic, usually under the skin of the upper arm. Very small quantities are used to start with, and the concentrations are increased week by week to avoid severe allergic reactions. The length of time and number of

DESENSITIZING SUFFERERS
If you are unable to avoid contact with a particular allergen, such as the family pet, desensitization is a possible option in some cases.

injections needed to complete the treatment vary. Small local reactions, consisting of a reddening of the skin at the injection site, are not infrequent, but these go away rapidly. Once the treatment is completed, booster shots can be given at varying intervals if the desensitization has been successful.

Desensitization for asthma is used only in a minority of patients, largely because of the fear of bad reactions but also because many doctors do not believe that this treatment is actually effective. If you wish to investigate further concerning whether this treatment may be helpful in your case, ask your doctor for a referral to an allergist. A list of specialist centers can be obtained from the American Academy of Allergy, Asthma, and Immunology (see Useful addresses, p.89).

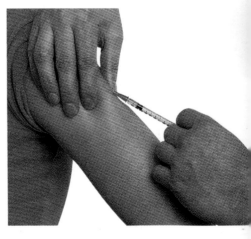

DESENSITIZATION
Desensitization involves a course of injections. Minute quantities of allergen are injected under the skin. The amount injected is gradually increased over a number of weeks until you are able to tolerate the allergen.

LIFE-THREATENING ASTHMA

Life-threatening asthma is a rare form of asthma. Patients suffer from sudden severe attacks, sometimes in spite of the fact that their asthma is generally under good control. Others who have a history of poorly controlled asthma can develop sudden severe attacks. These patients are often admitted to the hospital and are at increased risk of dying from their asthma.

Allergy seems to be more common in these patients, and sometimes their acute attacks follow inhaling or eating something to which they are allergic. Their asthma often puts a huge strain on both the patients and their families, and, psychological factors seem to be very important. Whether the asthma causes the psychological disturbance or vice versa is not clear.

Treatment is extremely difficult, and patients should be managed by pulmonary specialists with interest and expertise in the more severe forms of asthma.

ASPIRIN-SENSITIVE ASTHMA

Aspirin sensitivity occurs in about 5 percent of adult patients with asthma but is very rare in children. Very often these patients' skin tests are negative for allergens, and they may also suffer from recurring nasal polyps. If you are such a patient, you must avoid all aspirin-containing medications, including a wide range of arthritis formulas such as ibuprofen, diclofenac, and indomethacin. If you are not sure whether a particular drug might make your asthma worse, ask your doctor or pharmacist. Aspirin-sensitive asthmatic patients can die from unknowingly swallowing a preparation containing aspirin. Although the treatment usually involves avoidance, desensitization can also be achieved successfully. However, this particular treatment is available only in special clinics.

Desensitization for this form of asthma is done using small doses of aspirin that are administered orally. The patient is closely monitored at the hospital or clinic with repeated breathing tests for several hours after each dose. Although it is a time-consuming process, it is worthwhile for some patients.

NOCTURNAL ASTHMA

Nighttime asthma is often regarded as a particular type of asthma. In fact, waking up at night with asthma is an indication of asthma that is poorly controlled and

CHECK THE INGREDIENTS
If you are sensitive to aspirin, be sure to check with your doctor or pharmacist before taking any medication.

should be a warning signal for patients with any type of asthma. In most cases, appropriate treatment will overcome the problem, but in some patients it is more difficult to control.

In these patients, factors such as acid reflux (stomach acid coming back into the esophagus at night and causing irritation) may be a cause of nocturnal asthma and require treatment. Some drugs, such as theophyllines and the long-acting inhaled bronchodilators, are often helpful in controlling the symptoms of nocturnal asthma.

NIGHTTIME ASTHMA
People with asthma commonly have symptoms during the night. This may indicate that their asthma is poorly controlled.

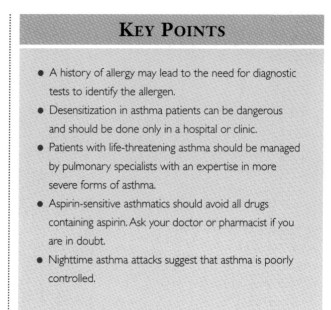

KEY POINTS

- A history of allergy may lead to the need for diagnostic tests to identify the allergen.
- Desensitization in asthma patients can be dangerous and should be done only in a hospital or clinic.
- Patients with life-threatening asthma should be managed by pulmonary specialists with an expertise in more severe forms of asthma.
- Aspirin-sensitive asthmatics should avoid all drugs containing aspirin. Ask your doctor or pharmacist if you are in doubt.
- Nighttime asthma attacks suggest that asthma is poorly controlled.

Occupational asthma

Asthma that develops as a result of exposure to a substance or substances in the workplace is known as occupational asthma.

The exposure to the substance may act as an inducer, and the offending substance may sensitize the patient to such an extent that further asthmatic reactions occur at every subsequent exposure. Alternatively, the substance may act as a trigger, precipitating attacks in patients who already have asthma that did not necessarily develop as a result of the exposure.

CAUSES

There are more than 200 known causes of occupational asthma. Many of them are obscure, but some occur in very familiar work environments. Causes of occupational asthma include epoxy resins, flour, and isocyanates, the hardener in paints used by car body paint sprayers.

A list of the more common substances causing occupational asthma is given on page 68, along with the jobs with which they are usually associated.

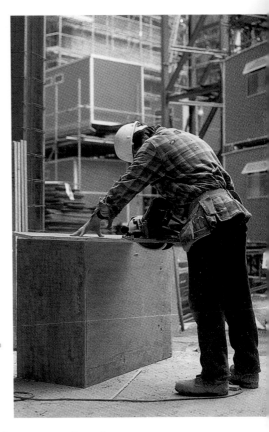

OCCUPATIONAL HAZARDS
Work that involves constant exposure to dust or another allergen can cause asthma in susceptible people. If protection is not possible, it may require a change of job.

Common Causes of Occupational Asthma

Some of the most common causes of occupational asthma are shown in this chart, together with the jobs in which you are most likely to encounter each substance.

CAUSES/SUBSTANCES	OCCUPATIONS
Isocyanates	Occupations involving paint, varnish, and some plastics
Colophony (Rosin)	Soldering
Animal urine	Laboratory workers, animal breeders
Epoxy resins	Occupations involving adhesives and varnishes
Flour	Baking or catering trades
Chromium	Tanning, electroplating
Enzymes	Detergent production, drug/food technology
Hardwood dusts	Millers, joiners, carpenters
Nickel	Electroplating
Dyes	Dye manufacturing
Antibiotics	Drug manufacturing
Grain mites	Farmers

COMMON OCCURRENCE

Occupational asthma may affect about 5 percent of asthmatics. However, this figure is approximate and is undoubtedly an underestimate of the true number. Since patients, employers, and doctors are often unaware of the possibility that occupational factors could be significant, many of these cases go undiagnosed. In some individuals, this oversight may be a problem because continued occupational exposure to certain substances can lead to irreversible changes in the airways.

DIAGNOSIS

The first clue comes from the patient's medical history. If your symptoms improve over the weekend or when you are away from work for longer periods, such as during vacations, something at work may be triggering your asthma. Not all those who give such a medical history have occupational asthma, but some who do not may end up with this diagnosis. However, such a history should prompt referral to a specialist for further tests.

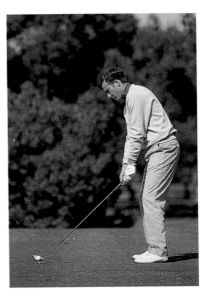

ABSENCE FROM WORK *Symptoms that improve during breaks from work, such as vacations, only to begin again on returning, suggest that something in the workplace may be the cause of a person's asthma.*

The specialist will ask you to record your peak flows regularly, perhaps as frequently as every two hours, to look for recognizable patterns of change in peak flow readings that would support the diagnosis.

Case History: **SPRAY-PAINT ALLERGY**

Brian was 32 years old. He had been working in the automobile industry for 10 years, ever since he left the Army, where he learned his trade. For the first four years Brian did various jobs around the factory, but he was switched to the paint shop at the age of 26. Although he smoked 10 to 15 cigarettes a day, his only problem up until to that time had been occasional bouts of winter bronchitis. During the winter of 1990, however, he had what he thought was another attack of bronchitis with coughing and wheezing, but on this occasion the symptoms persisted and began to wake him at night. He went to his doctor, who prescribed antibiotics and told him he had to stop smoking. However, the antibiotics had no effect, and Brian's wheezing began to be obvious after even modest exertion. The doctor thought that Brian might have asthma and treated him with some success shortly before Brian went away on vacation at Easter in 1991.

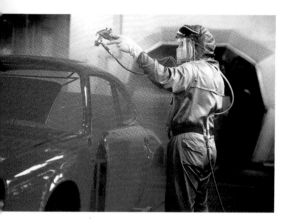

SPRAYING SAFELY
A ventilated hood offered enough protection from the offending paint allergen to prevent Brian's symptoms from recurring.

While he was away, Brian began to feel much better and even stopped using his inhalers. As soon as he went back to work, however, his asthma returned with a vengeance. Suspecting that Brian's improvement while he was away from work might indicate an occupational aspect to his asthma, his doctor referred him to a specialist. Serial peak flow readings showed the typical pattern of work-related asthma. Luckily, the firm for which Brian worked provided him with an effective protective hood. Since Brian started wearing the hood, his asthma has been easier to control, and, consequently, he has been able to continue work at his job.

CONFIRMING THE DIAGNOSIS

Occasionally, if there is still doubt about whether there is an occupational component to your asthma, you may be tested by an occupational medicine physician with the suspected substance under carefully supervised conditions. If you react when exposed to the suspected agent but not when exposed to another substance, the diagnosis will become clear. This is a time-consuming process because you may have to take a week off from work to undergo repeated series of breathing tests after differing exposures in a specially constructed laboratory.

THE PATIENT'S FUTURE

Some people are forced to leave their jobs because their asthma is too difficult to control while they are exposed. In many cases, management may be either unable or unwilling to improve workplace conditions. Some patients are repositioned within the company to a job at which exposure to the offending substance does not occur. Many, however, continue to be exposed, which may be acceptable in some cases if the asthma can be controlled by medication.

KEY POINTS

- Asthma symptoms that improve over the weekend or during vacations suggest an occupational cause.
- The clue usually comes from the history, but the diagnosis may need to be confirmed in the laboratory.

Complementary treatments

There is considerable interest in the role of alternative or complementary therapies in the treatment of asthma. This may be because some people are concerned about the side effects of conventional medical treatment and believe that natural substances are better for asthma than are drugs.

HEALING HERBS
The eucalyptus plant is used in herbal medicine to treat asthma.

Although virtually all of the available standard asthma treatments have been established in properly controlled trials of efficacy, only rarely have complementary approaches been assessed in this way. For example, since herbal medicines are not licensed by the Food and Drug Administration, the quality of these products may vary widely. As a result, many doctors are not enthusiastic about such forms of treatment. Yet complementary practitioners often quote anecdotal stories of benefit and maintain that consistent successes over many years show that this kind of treatment works. There may even be a polarization between those who believe that conventional medicine is the only suitable treatment and those who believe conventional treatment leaves much to be desired.

Complementary Therapies

*Claims of benefit from the treatment of asthma with complementary therapies
have rarely been assessed by clinical trials.*

ACUPUNCTURE

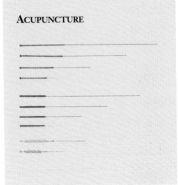

There is no doubt that acupuncture has found
more acceptance in conventional medical circles
than have many other forms of complementary
therapy, particularly in regard to pain relief. It is also
one of the few alternative approaches to asthma
treatment that has been tested in clinical trials.
Minor benefits have been shown in mild asthma,
but acupuncture has not been shown to be of great
help in patients with more severe symptoms.

HERBALISM

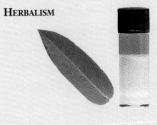

Herbalists often direct therapy at symptoms
rather than at the condition itself. If coughing is a
predominant symptom of asthma, treatment focuses
on specific attempts to reduce sputum production,
often with suggestions for dietary control.

HYPNOSIS

Some patients claim great benefits from hypnosis,
particularly in the way they are able to cope
with acute attacks or worsening asthma.
For those who believe in this approach,
it may be of help, but properly conducted
trials of its effects are as yet lacking.

Complementary Therapies (cont'd.)

HOMEOPATHY

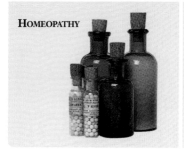

There are claims that homeopathic remedies for chronic asthma work, but there is little, if any, objective or scientific proof of these claims.

Nevertheless, there needs to be a holistic approach to the treatment of an asthmatic person. His or her beliefs need to be considered and discussed, and, where there are strong beliefs on both sides, compromises can be made. It must always be remembered that the aim is to control asthma or at least reduce it to a level that is acceptable for the patient.

Conventional therapy should remain the mainstay in the treatment of asthma. Patients should not suddenly stop conventional treatment and switch to an alternative therapy. Such abrupt changes have resulted in marked deterioration in some individuals.

KEY POINTS

- Complementary therapies may help some patients. Whether this is due to belief in the effectiveness of the alternative approach or to a direct effect on asthmatic airways has not been established.
- With the exception of acupuncture, the benefits of complementary approaches in the treatment of asthma have not adequately been tested in properly controlled trials.

The future

What does the future hold for the patient with asthma? First, there is no doubt that asthma is not going to disappear. It is very common, is likely to remain at current levels for the foreseeable future, and will continue to result in some deaths. Although this sounds very pessimistic, there are a number of potential developments that hold out hope to patients with asthma.

A FULL LIFE
With new drugs and treatments available, asthma sufferers can expect to lead a fairly normal, active life.

PREVENTION

It is likely that our ability to control exposure to allergens will improve in the coming years, and this will be especially important in the first five years of life, when sensitization to the house dust mite occurs. However, such control will require considerable effort on the part of the individual patient and, especially, the parents.

Doctors, for their part, have to come up with an even better package of control measures that is both practical and economical.

Other environmental control measures are needed, particularly a reduction in parental smoking, which is so significant in the development of asthma in children.

There are distinct signs that pollution control measures for cities and towns are now being adopted. These measures have improved air quality and could thereby lead to a reduction in the number of asthma attacks.

TREATMENT

Producing a new drug for any condition is a long and costly business, requiring stringent animal and human studies that have to satisfy the FDA that it is both useful and safe. What new drugs are being developed to help asthmatic patients in the near future?

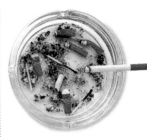

PARENTAL RESPONSIBILITY
Parents who smoke should give up the habit. Smoking has been proven to be instrumental in the development of childhood asthma.

NEW PILLS

Interestingly, some of the new drugs on the horizon are in pill form, as is the case with the leukotriene inhibitors (see p.42). Inhalers are often tricky to use effectively and are only rarely used as regularly as doctors would like to believe they are.

It is still unclear whether these new drugs, either inhaled or oral, will benefit all asthmatics. Certainly, they have the potential to make asthma control easier and more acceptable, with fewer side effects.

It is likely that, in the longer term, very specific treatments, perhaps aimed at particular groups of asthmatic patients, will become available. Whether these will be in inhalant or pill form will depend on many things, not the least of which will be the preferences of the patients themselves.

VACCINES

The possibility of being immunized against the allergy antibody, immunoglobulin E, as opposed to being desensitized to specific allergens is being investigated. This sounds attractive, but the medical profession is waiting to see if this therapy is safe, practical, and effective.

Immunization against viruses that most frequently cause asthma attacks – largely the common cold viruses, or rhinoviruses – may become a distinct possibility in the future once the appropriate vaccines become available. Again, trials will be necessary to prove that they can reduce attacks safely.

GENE THERAPY

Great strides are being made in unraveling the genetics of asthma, particularly with respect to allergy. Potentially, gene therapy could have a great effect on asthma, but there are many hurdles, both ethical and scientific, to be overcome. The reality of gene therapy is a long way off.

CONCLUSION

There is reason for optimism about the future for the asthmatic patient. Drugs with fewer side effects or, better still, improved ways of preventing asthma or asthma attacks will become available and will reduce the discomfort asthma sufferers endure today.

KEY POINTS

- New drugs are being tested that have the potential to make asthma control easier and more acceptable, with fewer side effects.
- Asthma will not be eradicated; however, attempts to prevent rather than treat asthma may be effective.

How to use your inhaler

How to Use the Metered Dose Inhaler

1 Remove the protective mouthpiece cover and shake the inhaler.
2 Exhale gently.
3 Put the mouthpiece in your mouth or in front of the lips and, at the start of a slow deep inspiration, press the canister down and continue to inhale deeply.
4 Hold your breath for 10 seconds or as long as possible.
5 Wait 30 seconds before taking another dose.

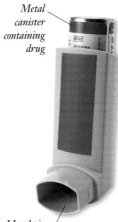

Metal canister containing drug

Mouthpiece

METERED DOSE INHALER

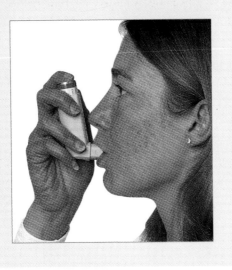

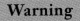

Warning

If in doubt, always seek professional advice.

Lever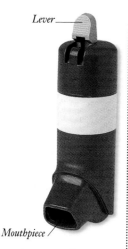

Mouthpiece

AUTOHALER DEVICE

How to Use the Autohaler Device

1 Remove the protective mouthpiece cover and shake the inhaler.
2 Hold the inhaler upright and push the lever up.
3 Exhale gently. Keep the inhaler upright, put the mouthpiece in your mouth, and close your lips around it. The air holes must not be blocked by your hand.
4 Inhale steadily through your mouth. DON'T stop breathing when the inhaler clicks but continue taking a very deep breath.
5 Hold your breath for about 10 seconds.

Note: The lever must be pushed up (on) before each dose and pushed down (off) afterward; otherwise, it will not operate.

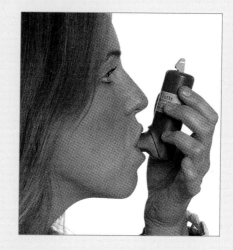

How to use the Diskus

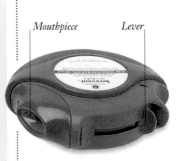

Mouthpiece   Lever

DISKUS

1 Hold the outer casing of the Diskus in one hand, with the mouthpiece toward you, while pushing the thumb grip away until a click is heard. This makes the dose available for inhalation and moves the dose counter ahead.

2 Holding the Diskus level, gently exhale away from the device, put the mouthpiece in your mouth, and suck in steadily and deeply.

3 Remove the Diskus from your mouth and hold your breath for about 10 seconds.

4 To close, slide thumb grip back toward you as far as it will go until it clicks.

5 For a second dose, repeat steps 1–4.

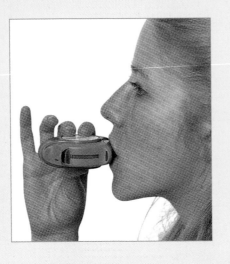

Warning

If in doubt always seek professional advice.

Grip

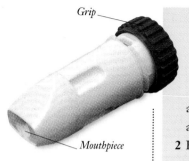

Mouthpiece

TURBOHALER

How to Use the Turbohaler

1 Unscrew and lift off the white cover. Hold the Turbohaler upright and twist the grip forward and backward as far as it will go. You should hear a click.

2 Exhale gently, put the mouthpiece between your lips, and inhale as deeply as possible. Even when a full dose is taken, there may be no taste.

3 Remove the Turbohaler from your mouth and hold your breath for about 10 seconds before exhaling. Replace the white cover.

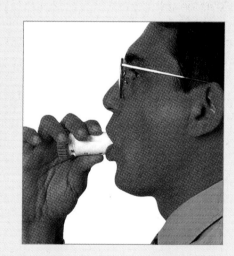

Warning

If in doubt, always seek professional advice.

How to Use the Diskhaler

To Load

1 Remove the mouthpiece cover. Remove the white tray by pulling it out gently and then squeezing the white ridges on either side until it slides out.
2 Put the foil disk – number side on the top – on the wheel and slide the tray back.
3 Holding the corners of the tray, slide the tray in and out to rotate the disk until an "8" shows in the window.

To Use

1 Keep the Diskhaler level and lift the rear of the lid as far up as it will go to pierce top and bottom of the foil disk. Close the lid.
2 Holding the Diskhaler level, exhale gently, put the mouthpiece (taking care not to cover the air holes on each side of it) in your mouth, and inhale deeply.
3 Remove the Diskhaler from your mouth and hold your breath for about 10 seconds. Slide the tray in and out to be ready for the next dose.

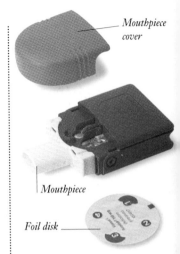

Mouthpiece cover

Mouthpiece

Foil disk

DISKHALER

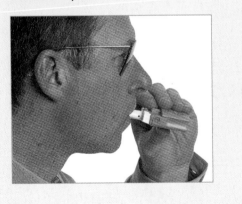

Warning

If in doubt, always seek professional advice.

Barrel

Mouthpiece

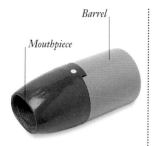

ROTAHALER

How to Use the Rotahaler

1 Hold the Rotahaler vertically and put the capsule into the "square" hole, colored end on top. Make sure the top of the Rotacap is level with the top of the hole. If there is already a Rotacap in the device, this one will be pushed into the shell.

2 Hold the Rotahaler horizontally; twist the barrel sharply forward and backward. This splits the capsule into two.

3 Exhale gently. Keep the Rotahaler level, put the mouthpiece between your lips and teeth, and inhale the powder quickly and deeply.

4 Remove the Rotahaler from your mouth and hold your breath for about 10 seconds.

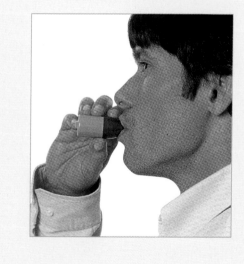

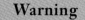

Warning

If in doubt, always seek professional advice.

How to Use the Spinhaler

1 Hold the Spinhaler upright with the mouthpiece downward and unscrew the barrel.
2 Put the colored end of a Spincap into the cup of the propeller, making sure it spins freely.
3 Screw the two parts together and move the gray sleeve up and down twice; this will pierce the Spincap.
4 Exhale gently, tilt your head back, put the Spinhaler into your mouth so that your lips touch the flange. Inhale quickly and deeply.
5 Remove the Spinhaler from your mouth, hold your breath for about 10 seconds, then exhale slowly.
6 If powder is left in the Spincap, repeat steps 4 and 5 until it is empty.

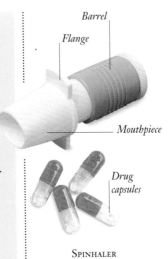

Barrel

Flange

Mouthpiece

Drug capsules

SPINHALER

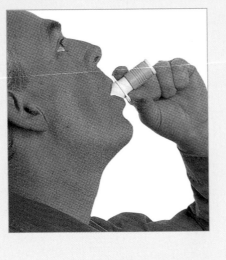

Warning

If in doubt, always seek professional advice.

Inhaler slot

Mouthpiece

VOLUME SPACER DEVICE

How to Use a Volume Spacer Device

Method for patients who can use the device without help:

1 Remove the cap, shake the inhaler, and insert it into the device.

2 Place the mouthpiece of the spacer in your mouth.

3 Press the canister once to release a dose of the drug.

4 Take a deep, slow breath.

5 Hold your breath for about 10 seconds, then exhale through the mouthpiece.

6 Inhale again, but without having first pressed the canister.

7 Remove the device from your mouth.

8 Wait about 30 seconds before taking a second dose.

The Multibreath Method

1 Follow steps 1–3 as detailed above.

2 Inhale and exhale ten times using normal-size breaths.

3 Remove the device from your mouth.

4 The next dose can be puffed into the spacer right away.

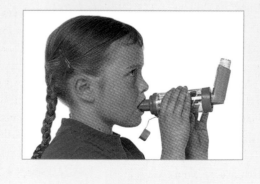

Warning

If in doubt, always seek professional advice.

Questions and answers

Will the asthma go away?

This is the question most commonly asked by parents about a child with asthma. Most children appear to outgrow asthma, often in their teens. This is not to say that the asthma disappears permanently, because a proportion of patients suffer a relapse later in life. In women, the relapse often occurs around the time of menopause.

Sometimes, the symptoms of recurrent asthma are different from those experienced as a child: wheezing is more common in childhood, and shortness of breath and chest tightness more common in adulthood.

Most people who develop asthma in adult life remain symptomatic to a greater or lesser degree for the rest of their lives. It is difficult to determine the proportion of those people who develop asthma in adulthood who stop having symptoms.

Will the asthma or the treatment of it damage the lungs?

The concern about long-term damage to the lungs is a real one. Asthma can lead to irreversible narrowing of the airways when the inflammation is not controlled. Similarly, patients who smoke and do not use their preventive inhaler regularly may develop severe, irreversible damage to their lungs.

Treatment for asthma itself does not damage the lungs, although steroid pills can cause many other side effects, as discussed before (see pp.58–59)

Considered overall, undertreated asthma is more likely to cause damage to the individual than the possible side effects of treatment are.

Will the treatment wear off?

The drug treatment for asthma does not wear off. If you find that your relief inhaler is becoming less effective, it is far more likely to be due to worsening asthma than to the drug itself having no effect. Perhaps the prescribed dose is too low, or, because the airways become narrower as the asthma worsens, less medicine may be reaching the lower airways.

If you find that your treatment is becoming less effective, it is essential that you see your doctor for reassessment. Taking a certain dose of an inhaled medication will not lead to a need for a progressively higher dose as the years go by.

Is asthma contagious?

No, it is not. Asthma is not an infectious disease and cannot be caught from another person.

Are nebulizers dangerous?

A nebulizer is a powerful means of delivering drugs to the lungs and is therefore used only by a patient with more severe asthma. Nevertheless, there are some patients using nebulizer therapy for whom other forms of treatment have not been fully explored. When used only for acute attacks, nebulizers can save lives and decrease hospital admissions. The danger comes when too much reliance is placed on the nebulizer. Instead of seeking medical help, the patient self-administers repeated nebulized doses. This can lead to a very severe, and even life-threatening episode which could have been avoided had the patient gone to the emergency room or contacted his or her doctor.

The need for regular nebulized therapy clearly indicates that the asthma is severe. Many patients will never be able to stop the treatment unless a better one is developed. In some cases, changes in circumstances, such as a move to a different area or removal from an occupational cause, can result in marked improvement in their asthma, and they may no longer need to use the nebulizer.

Again, as with other forms of inhaled therapy, using nebulized therapy under proper supervision does not mean that you will need higher and higher doses as the years go by. If that appears to be happening, it is more likely because the asthma itself is getting worse than because of an effect of the nebulized drug.

Useful addresses

Allergy and Asthma Network/Mothers of Asthmatics (AAN/MA)
Online: www.aanma.org
2751 Prosperity Avenue
Fairfax, VA 22031
Tel: (800) 878-4403
AAN/MA helps families control and overcome asthma. Resources include information on treatments, product development, and laws. It publishes a monthly newsletter and offers products at discounted prices.

American Academy of Allergy, Asthma, and Immunology (AAAAI)
Online: www.aaaai.org
611 East Wells Street
Milwaukee, WI 53202
Tel: (800) 822-2762
AAAAI is dedicated to the study and treatment of allergic diseases. The 24-hour, toll-free number can be used to obtain referrals to physicians throughout the country.

American College of Allergy and Immunology (ACAI)
Online: www.allergy.mcg.edu
85 West Algonquin Road
Arlington Heights, IL 60005
Tel: (800) 842-7777
Resources include booklets and books. The toll-free number can be used to obtain a list of allergists by state.

American Lung Association (ALA)
Online: www.lung.usa.org
1740 Broadway
New York, NY 10019
Tel: (800) LUNG-USA
ALA is concerned with all lung diseases, but a major focus of its research is asthma. Resources include publications such as *Asthma Magazine* and a family guide to asthma and research updates. ALA has nearly 250 local offices across the US.

Asthma and Allergy Foundation of America (AAFA)
Online: www.aafa.org
1125 Fifteenth Street NW
Washington, DC 20005
Tel: (800) 7-ASTHMA
Resources include pamphlets and books with an emphasis on children and adolescents, interactive CD-ROM games, and a bimonthly newsletter.

National Asthma Education and Prevention Program
Online: www.nhlbi.nih.gov
PO Box 30105
Bethesda, MD 20824
Tel: (301) 251-1222
This program, administered by the National Heart, Lung, and Blood Institute (NHLBI), educates patients and health care professionals about asthma. The Asthma Management Model System, at the website above, offers information on research, a database, and publications.

National Health Information Center (NHIC)
Online: http://nhic-nt.health.org
PO Box 1133
Washington, DC 20013
Tel: (800) 336-4797
NHIC, part of the Department of Health and Human Services, helps people locate information on health issues through referrals to organizations that can best answer their questions.

National Jewish Medical and Research Center
Online: www.njc.org
1400 Jackson Street
Denver, CO 80206
Tel: (800) 222-LUNG
This is the only medical and research center in the US devoted exclusively to respiratory and allergic diseases, including asthma.

Notes

Notes

Notes

Index

Acknowledgments

PUBLISHER'S ACKNOWLEDGMENTS

Dorling Kindersley Publishing, Inc. would like to thank the following for their help and participation in this project:

Managing Editor Stephanie Jackson; **Managing Art Editor** Nigel Duffield; **Editorial Assistance** Judit Z. Bodnar, Mary Lindsay, Nicola Munro, Irene Pavitt, Jennifer Quasha, Ashley Ren, Design Revolution, David Tombesi-Walton; **Design Assistance** Sarah Hall, Marianne Markham, Adam Powers, Design Revolution, Chris Walker; **DTP** Rachel Symons; **Production** Michelle Thomas, Elizabeth Cherry.

Consultancy Dr. Tony Smith, Dr. Sue Davidson, the Dartmouth-Hitchcock Medical Center, Hanover, NH, John Croteau, RPH, Enfield, NH; **Indexing** Indexing Specialists; **Administration** Christopher Gordon.

Organizations St. John's Ambulance, St. Andrew's Ambulance Organization, British Red Cross.

Photography (p.24, p.30, p.63, pp.79–85) Paul Mattock; **Illustrations** (p.8, p.17, p.45) ©Philip Wilson.

Picture Research Angela Anderson; **Picture Librarian** Charlotte Oster.

PICTURE CREDITS

The publisher would like to thank the following for their kind permission to reproduce their photographs. Every effort has been made to trace the copyright holders. Dorling Kindersley apologizes for any unintentional omissions and would be pleased, in any such cases, to add an acknowledgment in future editions.

Richard Gardner p.67; **Pictor Uniphoto** p.70.